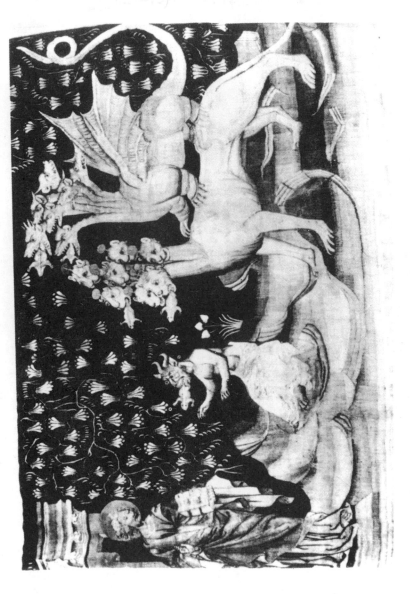

The many-headed dragon of terminal pain. Photograph of a medieval tapestry given to the authors by a patient who said: 'This is what my illness feels like to me.'

Living with Dying

A Guide to Palliative Care

Third Edition

CICELY SAUNDERS
MARY BAINES
and
ROBERT DUNLOP

OXFORD NEW YORK TOKYO
OXFORD UNIVERSITY PRESS
1995

PN
1146S

9505082

WB 310

Oxford University Press, Walton Street, Oxford OX2 6DP
Oxford New York
Athens Auckland Bangkok Bombay
Calcutta Cape Town Dar es Salaam Delhi
Florence Hong Kong Istanbul Karachi
Kuala Lumpur Madras Madrid Melbourne
Mexico City Nairobi Paris Singapore
Taipei Tokyo Toronto
and associated companies in
Berlin Ibadan

Oxford is a trade mark of Oxford University Press

Published in the United States
by Oxford University Press Inc., New York

A catalogue record for this book is available from the British Library

Library of Congress Cataloging in Publication Data
Saunders, Cicely M., Dame.
Living with dying : a guide to palliative care / Cicely
Saunders, Mary Baines, and Robert Dunlop. — 3rd ed.
Includes bibliographical references and index.
1. Terminal care. 2. Terminally ill—Psychology. I. Baines,
Mary. II. Dunlop, R. J. (Robert J.) III. Title.
R726.8.S28 1995 616'.029—dc20 94-38481
ISBN 0 19 262514 4

Typeset by Downdell, Oxford
Printed in Great Britain by
Redwood Books Ltd, Trowbridge, Wilts

A *foreword for people who are not experts in palliative care*

Looking after dying patients makes all of us feel uneasy and awkward at first. But no matter how nervous you feel to begin with, and no matter how little you think you know, if you are keen to do it, then reading this book will help you to do it well. I speak from personal experience: when I first became interested in the support of the terminally ill, I thought I was the only person in the world to feel anxious and ill at ease about it—and it was this book that helped me most. The second edition is even better than the first, and I am quite sure that you will find it clear, concise, practical, and useful—qualities that are not very common in many medical texts.

Now that I have become brave enough to ask other doctors and nurses how they felt when they started out in palliative care, I have found that almost everyone was nervous to some degree—but did not tell anyone else. I think there are many reasons for those feelings and perhaps it is worth thinking about them for a moment or two before reading the rest of this book.

I think that looking after a dying person seems (at first) to negate much of what we have learned in our training. Generally speaking, we are trained to recognize disease processes and to treat them—and, whenever possible, to cure them. It is not easy to be near someone who is dying and accept that your therapeutic efforts and endeavours should no longer be directed against the disease itself, but against the symptoms. It seems like defeatism—until you realize what a tremendous need there is for good symptom control, and how much you can achieve with your skill and support.

Facing (apparent) therapeutic failure is not the only problem. We also have to face the possibility that the patient may be angry and may blame us for the disease itself (blaming the messenger for the bad news), they may be tearful or depressed or exhibiting several of many reactions for which we have not been prepared in medical school, nursing college, or any other training course. We are likely to feel unskilled and inept—and often have a powerful urge to back out of the whole thing.

All I need to say is that those feelings are normal and that everyone has them when they start out. They fade with increasing experience. All you need to get you started is some factual knowledge and good communication skills.

I stress knowledge and communication because the first is useless without the second. It does not matter if you know the pharmacokinetics and plasma half-life of every opioid in the world, and the stereochemical structure of all the sub-types of endorphin receptor. If you do not know when the patient is experiencing pain, where it is, and how bad it is, you are not going to be able to help. The closer you get to understanding what the patient is feeling, the more effective you will be in supporting the patient and relieving the symptoms.

You will find that this book is full of practical hints and tips: let me tell you that they really work! Furthermore, nothing will increase your confidence in this difficult area like a little bit of success. This part of our job is one of the most difficult of all, but it is one of the most important and it has a huge impact on our patients and their families. You will find that this book will help you to help them.

1988   Robert Buckman
                                  (Medical Oncologist)

Preface

'It does not require a million pounds, or magic, but confidence that pain control is possible with detailed attention to a variety of therapeutic measures, coupled with that attitude which accepts the whole patient and his needs but sees him as a person.'

(Ford and Pincherle 1978)

We believe that the suggestions in this book can be applied wherever doctors find that their commitment to their patients *must* include treatment for terminal illness. They do not presuppose that the patient should be in a special hospice or palliative care unit, though this move may have to be made to solve complex physical and social problems. These are basic principles that can be interpreted and developed anywhere and the skills of a special team may never be needed.

Over the past three decades increasing attention has been given to the needs of patients with far advanced disease and their families, and the Hospice and Palliative Care Movements have developed in diverse ways. When St. Christopher's Hospice opened in 1967 as the first research and teaching hospice, its main aim was that tested knowledge should flow back into all branches of the National Health Service, as well as to the older homes and hospices to which it owed so great a debt. Earlier links with workers overseas had also encouraged hopes of extending even more widely, and these have been fulfilled. That there should now be specialist wards in general hospitals, and home and hospital teams working in consultation with the patient's own doctors, are in many ways more important developments than the growth of special units. Most important of all has been the general change of attitude to a more analytical and positive approach to the needs of a dying patient and his family. Anecdotal evidence is replaced increasingly by objective data as the scientific foundations of this branch of medicine are laid. The essentials of good management at this stage have been clarified and are now being widely discussed. Advances in this area of treatment (and it is still 'treatment', not some kind of soft option labelled 'care') are now likely to come from the traditional hospital setting as well as from the special units or teams. A patient, wherever he or she may be, should expect the same reasoned attention to suffering now as was received for the original diagnosis and treatment of the condition. The aim is no longer to cure but to give patients the chance to live to their fullest potential in physical ease and activity, with the assurance of personal relationships until they die.

The achievement we will be looking for will be the patient's own. It is an honour as well as an education to meet people making their way through such adversity with the courage and common sense they so often show. We may see this only as we come near to them and we have often found that the best way to do this is to develop skill in giving physical relief. We will not halt there if our patients give us the privilege of sharing their inner anguish. We may be able to do little to remove this but at least we can stand by them. Our hope is that this book will make it easier to do so.

Sydenham   C.S.
June 1994   M.B.
                                                 R.D.

Contents

1

Introduction

'I conceive it the office of the physician not only to restore the health but to mitigate pains and dolours; and not only when such mitigation may conduce to recovery but when it may serve to make a fair and easy passage.'

(Francis Bacon)

Health is more than the absence of disease or infirmity, it is the most effective use by an individual of the potential for living in physical, mental, and social well-being (World Health Organization 1946). The aim of the treatment of terminal disease is more than the mere absence of symptoms, it is that the patient and the family should live to the limits of their potential. The achievements to be looked for are not merely in physical ease and improvement, though these may be considerable, but in the use made of time given by these to deal with past problems, enjoy present opportunities, and probe future plans for the family who must live on afterwards.

Appropriate treatment

Doctors are committed to giving appropriate care to their patients, not to every treatment that may be technically possible: 'The prolongation of life should not itself constitute the exclusive aim of medical practice, which must be concerned equally with the relief of suffering.' (Council of Europe 1976).

The palliative approach may be relevant long before a patient nears the end of life. Attention to the person with a persistent disease, to the family whose life is disrupted by illness, as well as to the control of any distressing symptoms, should be given much earlier, while active treatment is still being pursued. Palliative medicine has been a recognized specialty in the United Kingdom since 1987 with the definition, 'The study and management of patients with active, progressive, far advanced disease, for whom the prognosis is limited and the focus of care is the quality of life.' Although no specific pathology is mentioned, most of the focus of the past two to three decades has been upon the total care of the person with far advanced cancer but much of what follows in this book should be seen as potentially relevant to people with other diagnoses (see p. 9). What is being researched and taught by the hospice and palliative care teams has a widening relevance.

Terminal care itself refers to the management of patients in whom the advent of death is felt to be certain and not too far off and for whom medical effort has turned away from (active) therapy and become concentrated on the relief of symptoms and the support of both patient and family. Many diseases have a terminal phase and patients suffering from them need treatment suited to their condition at that time. Continuity of care with appropriate treatments in series may be indicated as the disease progresses, together with a readiness to review both diagnosis and prognosis. As noted above, skilled control of the problems of advanced and terminal disease does not necessarily have to wait until all other treatment is abandoned; its successful use may indeed make that treatment more effective. When the clinician is involved with both chemotherapy and with the control of pain and nausea, it will be easier to recognize diminishing returns to the former and to discontinue it without any member of the team or family feeling that now no treatment is being given. Doctors, however, have often been unwilling to make such a judgement except in the various forms of malignant disease. These may have a comparatively long terminal phase, needing much skill and support if relief is to be given.

On making decisions

When it is appreciated that palliative care entail skilful and effective treatment and that unexpected remissions may still occur, doctors find it less difficult to discontinue active therapy. Palliative care to combat persistent disease is often rigorous but it may give good returns in active living or making curative treatment possible once again. If it is no longer effective the alternative is not merely custodial care. During the past decades it has become clear that to practise competent palliative medicine is both demanding and rewarding. It may give not only added quality to the life remaining but also, at times, add considerably to its length. For example, during the first 14 years of St. Christopher's practice 32 of the 1179 patients who were admitted for terminal care for cancer of the breast with widespread metastases enjoyed lives of good quality at home for one to six years after their presenting symptoms had been controlled, while 31 lived for between six months and a year. Their further care was shared between the original treating hospital and the hospice, wherever this was appropriate. Symptom control alone or further radiotherapy, chemotherapy, or hormone therapy made this possible, and much of the time was spent at home.

These two aims must be balanced, as the physician tries to act in the best interests of each patient. Ethical dilemmas are usually most satisfactorily considered in the context of particular situations. The risks, pain, likelihood of success, anticipated results, and side-effects are assessed for each patient. Not only physical but psychological and social aspects have to be considered and there must be opportunity to discuss the complex issues raised with all the staff involved. Although at times a 'trial of treatment', such as high-dose steroids for a patient with cerebral metastases, is indicated it should be remembered that it may be easier to withhold possible treatments than it is to withdraw them once they have been instituted. The patient (if possible) and the family should still maintain their right to fully informed consent and be able to choose or refuse particular courses of action. A meeting with all those involved, together with some of the professional team, may help greatly in giving accurate information and clarifying the issues. The use of the words 'ordinary' and 'extraordinary means', with the understanding that neither doctor nor patient need be committed to the latter (Pius XII 1957), does not excuse the doctor from going through an often complex process of deliberation to find what exactly they should mean for an individual patient. It has been suggested that when the actual criteria of decisions are specified the use of these words becomes redundant and may be omitted.

Patients have the right to refuse treatment and to have their choices respected, provided they are mature and lucid. If they are unconscious, a document drawn up previously giving general wishes, often described as a 'Living Will', may give the clinician some guidance as judgement is made. Patients' relatives have no right to make decisions on their behalf unless they are incompetent. They may act only according to what are now considered to be the best interests of the patient and should be helped to consider what these are by discussion with the different members of the professional team. The discussion of sharing truth so that truly informed consent can be considered, and plans and farewells made, is dealt with in the later section on mental pain.

Death with dignity

To accept a situation when treatment is directed to the relief of symptoms and the alleviation of general distress does not mean an implicit 'there is nothing more we can do' but an explicit 'everything possible is being done'. Our concern and interest in this field brings us to the dying person with ever-renewed concern and a positive attitude that is often transferred without words: 'It can do much to lift the feeling of helplessness from the situation and help the patient to die with a sense of worth to the end' (Vanderpool 1978). Nothing could undermine this more than any form of legalized deliberate ending of life.

Vanderpool and others have come to consider that, although popular, the phrase 'death with dignity' is used with such different interpretations that it is better abandoned. It suffers from a dangerous ambiguity, and serves to mask three quite distinct demands.

1. That the individual should in principle be free to determine whether he or she shall live or die and that, in the event of choosing to die, he or she should be entitled to be assisted in so doing by the medical profession, except in so far as rights are limited in the general interest.
2. That a doctor should, with the patient's consent, be free, under certain safeguards, to end the patient's life in cases (if there are such) where it is medically impossible to control the pain.
3. That (i) a patient *in extremis* should not be subjected to troublesome treatments which cannot restore that patient to health; and (ii) doctors may use drugs to control pain even at the risk of shortening life.

Point 3 does not entail euthanasia at all, for it does not entail deliberately killing the patient. Point 1 entails euthanasia on a different basis from Point 2 and on a larger scale. An expression which suffers from this degree of ambiguity is dangerously unsuitable for use in serious discussion.

Euthanasia

The doctor may not embark on any conduct with the primary intention of causing the patient's death, and if a terminally ill patient expresses a desire to commit suicide a doctor may not in law facilitate the suicide (Suicide Act 1961)—to do so would be a criminal offence. The doctor cannot respond to similar suggestions by the family to act deliberately to end life. Effective therapy and adequate explanations should dispel the misunderstandings that doctors are committed to prolonging life whatever its quality and that the only way to a peaceful dying is by a deliberate overdose. To ease the pains of death has always been one of the commitments of medical practice and if, to ease suffering, a doctor must take measures which may hasten death, this is permissible provided that the doctor's aim is only the relief of pain or other distress (BMA 1988). This reflects the so-called double effect theory and was incorporated into English law in one of the few decided cases in this area (Rex *v.* Bodkin Adams 1957). In his summing up Judge Devlin said '. . . the proper medical treatment that is administered and that has an incidental effect on determining the exact moment of death is not the cause of death in any sensible use of the term' (Devlin 1985).

The House of Lords Select Committee on Medical Ethics published its report early in 1994. It emphasized 'that the right to refuse medical treatment is far removed from the right to request assistance in dying'. Although the Committee had listened to much evidence of actual or anticipated suffering, they wrote 'we do not believe these arguments are sufficient reason to weaken society's prohibition of intentional killing. That prohibition is the cornerstone of law and order. It protects each of us impartially, embodying the belief that all are equal. . . . We believe that the issue of euthanasia is one in which the interest of the individual cannot be separated from the interest of society as a whole'.

They also strongly commended the development and growth of palliative care services—in hospices, in hospitals, and in the community, and recommended still more research and training in this field.

Everything must be done to develop better symptom control for the difficult problems remaining, to spread the knowledge already gained more widely and to desist from inappropriate measures that only serve to prolong or even increase distress. Above all, people with advanced disease and disability need the level of care and communication from those around them that comes from commitment to their individual worth.

Home care

Most cancer patients want to die at home. However, almost 80 per cent end up dying in hospitals, emphasizing how difficult home care is. There are several factors which result in hospital admission including uncontrolled symptoms especially pain, physical exhaustion of the carer, and the emotional burden caused by lack of information, the sense of responsibility if something goes wrong, and the feeling that health professionals could provide better care. Palliative care delivered in the home setting, usually by a multidisciplinary team which includes the general practitioner and district nurses, can address these factors and significantly increase the number who die at home.

Ideally, support and advice should be available to the patient and family 24 hours daily and seven days a week. General practitioners find that giving their home telephone number to the family is rarely abused and brings great comfort. Sufficient time should be set aside for visits to allow the patient and family to talk about their fears. The Macmillan or hospice home care nurse can facilitate this. Some doctors find it hard to visit if there are no specific medical problems but families value the contact.

Some fears will be unfounded and appropriate information will reassure. Appropriate concerns should be acknowledged, contingency plans can then be devised and practised. For example, in the event of a fall the patient should be made comfortable before helpful neighbours or family or the ambulance are contacted to help the person back into bed. Medications such as analgesics and anti-emetics can be left in the house with written instructions. Never underestimate the capabilities of patients and families; even the very distressing problem of massive haemorrhage from a fungating head and neck tumour can be planned for with many families.

When death is obviously approaching, information about the process of dying can be helpful. Families should be reassured that increasing sleepiness and possible confusion are due to the disease and not to medication. Forewarning them about the reduced food and fluid intake will also relieve significant distress. Other signs may include incontinence, irregular and 'rattling' breathing, skin mottling, and cool peripheries. The point of death should be described: the person stops breathing and cannot be roused. The family should be given advice about who to contact and they often need reassurance that it is not necessary to call for an ambulance or the police.

Clearly, not every person can or should die at home. Families often feel guilty if they cannot manage; they will need support and confirmation. Even if a positive decision has been made to stay at home, it will often help the family if an alternative has been discussed. Early referral to district nursing and hospice home care services will reduce the physical burden of care but a respite admission may be necessary if the illness is protracted. When the person is dying at home, the presence of a nurse in the house overnight can be very supportive.

Whatever the outcome, encouragement and praise for the

family is essential. Many families start out feeling afraid and helpless, the act of caring can be very draining, but there is nothing so satisfying as sharing with the family as they look back and say, with some pride, 'We didn't think we could have managed that'.

Palliative care for non-malignant conditions

Cancer only accounts for about 25 per cent of all deaths. It remains the most feared diagnosis, tending to overshadow the fact that many of the people who die from non-malignant conditions have to contend with distressing physical symptoms, psychosocial problems, and spiritual anguish. Likewise, their families have to cope with the physical demands of caring, the helplessness of having to watch a loved one suffering, and the fears and sadness that accompany a terminal illness.

Although the options for treating non-malignant diseases are increasing all the time, many patients will reach a point where these treatments produce little benefit, for example in severe cardiac or respiratory failure, or uraemia when transplantation or dialysis is not possible. There are still many diseases, such as the progressive neurological disorders, for which no specific treatments exist. Using Motor Neurone Disease (MND) as a model, St. Christopher's Hospice has demonstrated that the principles of palliative care can be successfully applied to patients with diseases other than cancer (O'Brien *et al.* 1992). For example, morphine can safely be used to relieve the pain and fear of choking that may occur in this disease. Symptom control for non-cancer conditions follows the same general principles as for cancer. Specifically ask about any symptom which distresses the patient, not just the symptoms usually associated with the illness. Doctors often ask patients with heart failure about paroxysmal nocturnal dyspnoea and orthopnoea but fail to ask about or treat nausea, dry mouth, constipation, and the pain associated with congestion. Diligence about regular prescribing and review is also necessary, especially because the doses and dosing frequencies for analgesics, anti-emetics, and other palliative treatments will often need modification if there is severe organ failure. For example, oral morphine must be given less frequently in patients with uraemia, cirrhosis, or congestive cardiac failure; hyoscine should be avoided in renal failure.

The prognosis of many non-malignant conditions can be more difficult to estimate. Even so, it is still possible to encourage people to share fears about the future and concerns for their loved ones. This is particularly important when the patient deteriorates quickly, as is often the case in the acute hospital setting. All too often the needs of relatives are overlooked, especially the need for information about the condition of the patient. The family usually does not ask because they will be a bother to the doctor or the nurses. Health professionals should always make the effort to speak to the relatives, even a short contact will be greatly appreciated.

Community care is often provided by families supported by the primary health care team and other community-based services. Palliative care services are rarely involved but hospices can be a valuable source of advice about symptom management. Some hospice programmes, nursing homes, and hospital-based geriatric services will provide respite admissions to help ease the physical burden of care on relatives.

2

Terminal pain

The greatest fear of the dying and their families is the fear of pain. Sadly, this fear has often been justified. Terminal pain is frequently treated ineptly and the public myth that death from cancer involves unremitting distress is perpetuated. The statement 'I'm waiting for the pain to start' continues to be heard.

There are many reasons why terminal pain has been so poorly controlled. Until recently, the care of the dying has rarely been included in the training of doctors and nurses. With a few notable exceptions, medical and surgical textbooks have ignored the problems of pain control. In addition, there are misconceptions concerning the use of strong analgesics with a widespread fear of 'addiction'. In many parts of the world, the essential drugs are not available, due to government prohibition, medical reluctance, or inadequate finance.

However, the vast majority of patients dying with cancer and other diseases can be given good pain relief with the use of appropriate analgesics, adjuvant medication, and measures such as radiotherapy and nerve blocks. This relief can be sustained over long periods without impairment of the patient's alertness or personality and thus the quality of life can be maintained until the end.

Nature of terminal pain

A series of pictures painted by St. Christopher's patients illustrated how they saw the pain with which they presented. The feeling of being impaled by a red-hot nail, of being totally isolated from the world by the encircling 'muscles of tension' with nothing but the hypodermic to pierce through them, the sudden jabs on movement, and the implacable heaviness of pain were all illustrated vividly. So too was the conviction that one is no better than some kind of scrap heap or exists at the mercy of the demolition squad, suffering blow after blow, as in the drawing by Mrs E. S. These paintings express feelings that are common to many patients dying of cancer. They show, in a visual way, the fact that pain comprises both the unpleasant sensation and the emotional reaction to it. Pain is a somatopsychic experience.

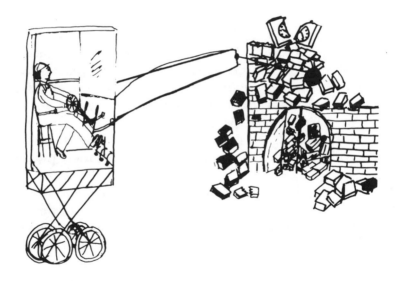

A patient (Mrs E. S.) draws the feeling of being constantly at the mercy of some kind of demolition squad.

The chronic pain of cancer is quite unlike the acute pain of trauma or the resolving pain of the postoperative period. These pains are easily understood, and even borne, when recovery is expected in a short time.

Cancer pain can appear to be unending, except by death. It is usually constant, worsening in severity, and associated with other unpleasant physical symptoms such as anorexia, vomiting, or dyspnoea.

Psychological factors greatly influence the perception of pain in terminal illness. Depression, anxiety, loneliness, and boredom will all lower the pain threshold. Such suffering is often termed 'Total Pain' and described as having physical, emotional, social, and spiritual components (Chapter 6). Unless these are all addressed the likelihood of successful pain control is small.

Prevalence

The World Health Organization (WHO) estimates that between 30 per cent and 50 per cent of cancer patients experience pain or are being treated for it. This percentage rises as the disease advances and about 70 per cent of those with advanced cancer suffer significant pain.

It is impossible to generalize about the degree of pain relief obtained but the situation has improved greatly over the last few years. This change is due to the increased impact of hospices, pain clinics, and palliative medicine services and to the initiative of the WHO Cancer Pain Relief Programme. This has provided guidelines for pain management and encouraged governments to make oral morphine available to all who need it (World Health Organization 1990).

Types of pain

Direct tumour involvement is the most common cause of pain in cancer patients. In most cases the pain is nociceptive, in that it is caused by mechanical or chemical stimuli in bone, viscera, etc. and conducted along intact somatosensory pathways. However, a significant proportion of cancer pain is neuropathic, caused by damage in the central or peripheral nervous system.

Some common cancer pains are as follows:

- Bone pain. Certain bone metastases produce prostaglandins which sensitize nociceptors and lead to pain. The pain is usually associated with local tenderness and is exacerbated by movement.
- Neuropathic pain. This often occurs with tumour infiltration of the brachial plexus or lumbar plexus, or injury to nerve roots due to vertebral metastases. However, neuropathic pain can occur with many other types of damage to the central or peripheral nervous system and therefore many further pain syndromes occur. Nerve pain is felt in the appropriate dermatome; it is often described as 'burning' or 'shooting' and is associated with motor, sensory, or autonomic changes.
- Visceral pain. This is due to tumour involving abdominal or pelvic organs.
- Lymphoedema. This occasionally follows surgery and radiotherapy; more often it is due to recurrent tumour.
- Intestinal colic from constipation or malignant obstruction.
- Headaches from raised intracranial pressure.

A significant proportion of the pain experienced by patients with advanced cancer is due to a non-malignant cause. Examples are as follows:

- Pain associated with cancer treatment. A thoracotomy scar may continue to be painful for months or years after surgery. Radiation therapy can cause immediate problems such as oesophagitis or long-term problems such as radiation fibrosis.

- Pain caused by debility. Patients with terminal disease are often bed or chairbound and develop the aches and pains of the immobile. Constipation is common, bedsores can develop rapidly as can thrush infections of the mouth.
- Other painful diseases. Elderly patients often have other painful conditions, such as arthritis or piles.

Clinical assessment of pain

Terminal pain, or indeed any other symptom, should be approached as an illness in itself, one that will respond to rationally based treatment.

A careful history of the pain is necessary. This should include site(s), severity, duration, exacerbating and relieving factors, interference with daily living, response to previous treatment, and a verbatim description such as 'like a red-hot poker' or 'painful pins and needles'. If possible, a body chart should be filled in by the doctor (or nurse) and patient together. The physical examination which follows should note any motor or sensory changes or local tenderness. The psychological state of the patient should be assessed, especially noting any evidence of depression. It is helpful to meet members of the family as well, they will often give additional information about the pain and its impact on the patient.

If the results of such a history and clinical examination are combined with the knowledge of pain mechanisms, it is usually possible to diagnose the cause of pain or pains. Sometimes further investigations are helpful but these may be impracticable in the very ill patient.

Management of pain

Treatment for pain should be started immediately, based on the presumptive diagnosis of its cause. Sometimes the response to treatment will make the diagnosis clearer or allow further investigations to be done. Occasionally the patient is too confused or ill for a full assessment to be made and, in this situation, adequate analgesia must be given without delay. For most patients, a combination of the following will be required:

- Analgesic drugs
- Adjuvant analgesic drugs
- Psychological and emotional support
- Palliative radiotherapy
- Anaesthetic techniques

The last two methods should always be considered (see Chapter 4), but in the majority of terminally ill patients the correct treatment is with the skilled use of drugs and the support of patient and family (see Chapters 3, 4 and 6).

Continual reassessment of the patient's pain is required as new pains develop and old pains alter in their severity and response to treatment.

3

The use of analgesics

While there is no need to resort automatically to strong analgesics when a patient approaches the terminal stages of his illness, pain must be relieved as soon as it becomes a matter for complaint. This complaint may have to be elicited, for these patients often underestimate the interest of others in their pain or the possibility of relief.

The criteria for giving analgesia, and especially the opioids, is the presence of pain—not the expected length of life. Many patients and families continue to fear that if morphine is started early it will 'lose its effect'. The reverse is nearer the truth, for good pain control throughout a terminal illness makes the use of high level opioids less likely. The really intractable pain, seen occasionally at the end of life, is often preceded by months of inadequate control leading to depression, anger, and fear.

Mild pain

Paracetamol and aspirin are the two common non-opioid analgesics. Both drugs are antipyretic, but aspirin alone has an anti-inflammatory effect. Paracetamol, 1000 mg 4–6-hourly, is recommended for the treatment of mild pain (maximum dose 4 g daily). This drug has fewer side-effects than aspirin, 600 mg 4-hourly, which should be reserved for pains in which its anti-inflammatory effect is required.

Moderate pain

Unfortunately, the majority of patients with malignant pain do not respond to paracetamol or aspirin. A change in medication is required and there are two possibilities:

- Weak opioid. This can be given in combination with a non-opioid, e.g. dextropropoxyphene and paracetamol (coproxamol) 2 tablets, 4-hourly, or alone as codeine 30–60 mg 4-hourly.
- Low dose of a strong opioid, e.g. morphine 5–10 mg 4-hourly.

The first option is recommended by the World Health Organization (1990) and may, indeed, be the only possible treatment in parts of the world where strong opioids are difficult to obtain ·or unavailable. However, the choice will usually depend on other factors: the expected rate in increase in severity of pain, the patient's wishes and the prognosis. With escalating pain or a very sick patient it is advisable to change directly from paracetamol or aspirin to morphine. Appropriate adjuvant therapy (Chapters 2 and 4) should be continued.

Moderate or severe pain

At St. Christopher's Hospice, morphine is the drug of choice for the management of moderate or severe pain caused by advanced cancer. The use of morphine will be considered in detail. Alternatives are shown in Table 1. These can be used for the rare cases of morphine intolerance or for the patient with a persistent morphine phobia.

Table 1 Alternatives to oral morphine

Name	Dose interval	Tablet	Morphine equivalent (as 4-hourly solution)	Comment
Buprenorphine	8 hours	0.2 mg 8-hourly	7 mg	Given sublingually. Probable ceiling dose at 4 mg/24 hours.
Dextromoramide	2 hours	5 mg (and 10 mg)	15 mg (peak effect)	Too short acting for regular use.
Methadone	8–12 hours	5 mg	7.5 mg single dose	Long plasma half-life. Requires careful titration (see p. 24)
Oxycodone	8 hours	30 mg suppository 8-hourly	15 mg	Preferred analgesic suppository.
Pethidine	2–3 hours	50 mg	5 mg	Weak oral analgesic. Short acting. Hyperexcitability with repeated doses.
Phenazocine	8 hours	5 mg 8-hourly	20 mg	Useful alternative to morphine. Sublingual administration.

Morphine

Pharmacology

Morphine is well absorbed when given by mouth, mainly in the proximal small bowel. Buccal and rectal absorption are more variable. Metabolism occurs mainly in the liver where morphine is broken down into glucuronides and it is in this form that most renal excretion occurs. One of the metabolites, morphine-6-glucuronide is much more potent than morphine itself and the analgesic effect of morphine results from the combined effects of morphine and this active metabolite. The plasma half-life of morphine and morphine-6-glucuronide is about 3 hours, so morphine should be given 4-hourly to maintain a satisfactory plasma level (unless a sustained release preparation is used).

Preparations and routes of administration

The oral route is the preferred method for giving morphine. If the patient is unable to tolerate this, a change is normally made to a subcutaneous infusion. Other routes may be indicated in particular circumstances.

Oral

1. Morphine sulphate tablet or solution, given 4-hourly.
2. Controlled release morphine tablet (MST or Oramorph SR) or granules (MST), given 12-hourly.

Injection

Morphine sulphate injections are widely available but if diamorphine is allowed (as in the UK) this is preferred because of its greater solubility. Both morphine and diamorphine have a ratio of injected dose:oral dose of 1:3 (with repeated administration).

1. Continuous subcutaneous infusion. A portable battery operated syringe driver or similar device is used and the drugs loaded every 24 hours. This route is used if pain is associated with severe vomiting, dysphagia, or if the patient is semiconscious. The opioid is usually combined with anti-emetic or sedative drugs. There is no evidence that this route improves pain control.

2. Subcutaneous or intramuscular bolus. These may be used in an emergency and 4-hourly injections may be needed in the last days of life if titration of dose is difficult.

3. Epidural morphine. This is given 12-hourly, or by infusion. The ratio of epidural dose:oral dose is 1:10. The main indication is for patients whose pain has been found to be opioid sensitive but who have unacceptable side-effects from systemic opioids. Morphine is often combined with a local anaesthetic (see Chapter 4).

Rectal

1. Morphine suppositories, 15 mg and 30 mg are available. The dose is the same as for oral morphine and needs to be given 4-hourly.

2. Controlled release morphine tablets have been given rectally but the absorption of morphine may be unpredictable.

Clinical use of morphine

Regular giving and individual dosage

The most rapid control of pain is obtained by the use of immediate release morphine, either in tablet or elixir form. This should be given 4-hourly to maintain a relatively constant blood level. The dose should be increased every 24 hours by 30%–50% increments until pain relief is obtained. Top-up doses for breakthrough pain should be allowed as often as necessary. Once pain control is achieved, most patients will prefer to change to controlled release morphine tablets 12-hourly for convenience of administration.

This pattern of morphine administration, with a careful titration of dose against the patient's pain, automatically allows for individual variation in age, weight, hepatic and renal function. The same methods have been used satisfactorily in children.

Dose range

If pain has escaped control by regular paracetamol, then 5 mg of morphine 4-hourly is suggested. A 10 mg dose 4-hourly is usually needed if the patient has been receiving regular co-proxamol or a similar weak opioid. However, the dose can be safely increased, as necessary. Most patients require less than 200 mg daily, but occasionally 1000 mg daily, or even higher, is needed.

When the correct dose has been found it will often remain at that level for weeks or months. Occasionally the dose can be reduced, following radiotherapy, a nerve block, or simply a lessening of anxiety. Sometimes, the level of analgesia needs to be steadily increased, this is usually due to progression of the disease.

Not 'p.r.n.'

Giving morphine solely 'on demand' or p.r.n. is indefensible. It puts the onus to ask on the patient who will often wait in pain, hoping that it will improve and not wanting to be a nuisance. Even if he or she is in control and takes analgesia as soon as the pain emerges, the drug will take time to be absorbed and so there is a constant reminder of pain and the cancer causing it. One of the many pleasures of working in a hospice is the expression of surprise seen when some patients are asked 'Have you any pain?' With regular analgesia they have been able to forget pain and concentrate on enjoying the life that is left.

Patient-controlled analgesia

This is a method of giving opioids intravenously or subcutaneously and allowing patients to titrate their own analgesic requirements, giving themselves medication when the pain occurs. This method has been used, with great benefit, for the control of postoperative pain. The disadvantage with cancer patients is that it regularly focuses their thoughts on the pain which occurs, the decision they must make about analgesia, and, inevitably, on the underlying disease. A further problem is that the pumps for patient-controlled analgesia are usually expensive and sophisticated.

Problems with morphine

- *Nausea and vomiting.* About one third of patients feel nauseated on starting morphine, so an anti-emetic such as metoclopramide should be given to prevent this; it can usually be stopped after a week.
- *Constipation.* This should be anticipated and laxatives prescribed routinely. (See p. 37.)
- *Sedation.* This normally resolves within a few days.
- *Respiratory depression.* This rarely presents a problem if the oral morphine dose is titrated carefully against the patient's pain, for pain is a respiratory stimulant. Tolerance to respiratory depression develops rapidly so that high doses of morphine can be used, if necessary, without significant risk.

- *Myoclonic jerks*. A reduction in morphine dose is needed if these are severe. If the pain then recurs, an alternative strong opioid should be considered.
- *Tolerance*. Many people fear that the dose of morphine will need to be increased steadily to produce the same effect. This makes some doctors reluctant to prescribe morphine 'too soon' and some patients are unwilling to take it. In fact, tolerance is a minor problem. When an increasing dose of morphine is needed this is usually due to increased pain from the advancing malignancy.
- *Physical dependence*. This does develop with regular morphine administration, but it is not a clinical problem. If pain lessens it is possible to reduce the dose of morphine gradually without producing withdrawal symptoms.
- *Psychological dependence*. Experience has shown that this rarely, if ever, occurs in cancer patients receiving morphine for cancer pain. With regular administration, usually of an oral drug, there is no rapid rise in blood level giving the 'high' which the addict craves.

The use of methadone

Methadone has an average plasma half-life of 24 hours, whereas the duration of analgesia is considerably shorter. Repeated doses can lead to considerable drug accumulation with resultant sedation and confusion. This has led to the use of methadone being discouraged. However, methadone is cheap and widely available and there is evidence that a few patients whose pain has become 'morphine non-responsive' are helped by methadone. The following methods are suggested if methadone is used.

The opioid-naive patient should be given methadone 5 mg, this dose is repeated every 30 minutes until pain control is achieved. No further analgesia is given until the pain begins to return, when the same method is repeated twice over. A simple calculation will then determine the daily dose required and half of this should be given 12-hourly.

When changing from morphine to methadone, the daily dose of morphine should be calculated and one tenth of the dose of methadone given. This dose is repeated as needed, but not more frequently than 3-hourly. A similar procedure is then followed as for the opioid-naive patient, and a twice daily dose calculated.

Continual reassessment

Terminal illness is progressive, not static. Cancer pain usually increases in intensity as the tumour enlarges in size, the patient weakens and anxieties multiply. New pains often emerge, sometimes directly due to the malignant process, but often due to associated complaints such as constipation or indigestion. The relief of one pain by a local measure may allow another pain to surface.

The successful treatment of cancer pain must therefore involve continual reassessment. In practice, this involves hourly monitoring of a hospitalized patient in severe pain. If pain is mild to moderate it is reasonable to assess the response to treatment every one or two days. Most patients at home will be contacted once or twice a week but should be told to report if pain alters or increases.

4

Adjuvant therapy in pain control

The control of pain in advanced cancer does not involve simply the use of analgesics. Radiotherapy and nerve blocks are indicated for a proportion of patients and many others will benefit from the use of adjuvant drugs. Such treatment may mean that opioids are not required at all, but more often the pain is controlled with a lower dose of morphine and fewer side-effects.

Palliative radiotherapy

Radiotherapy may be helpful during the last weeks of a patient's life, provided it is applied skilfully. It must be given without delay, with the minimum number of treatments, and its benefit must have been carefully balanced against the price the patient has to pay in terms of the time and trouble entailed. Its aim is to relieve symptoms with the lowest possible dose in the fewest possible treatments and with the minimum of side-effects. Regular liaison with the local radiotherapist is essential for any doctor caring for the terminally ill.

The most common indication for radiotherapy is the development of a painful bony metastasis. Worthwhile pain relief is achieved in 80 per cent of patients (50 per cent complete, 30 per cent partial). Price *et al.* (1986) in an important randomized prospective study, compared the pain relief from a single treatment of 8 Gy with a dose of 30 Gy in ten fractions over two weeks. There was no difference in the duration or degree of pain relief, or in morbidity.

Where there are generalized pains due to widespread bony metastases, hemibody irradiation may be indicated. Either the upper or lower half is irradiated in a single treatment of 6–8 Gy. Pain relief in 80 per cent of patients is reported. The development of spinal cord compression is an indication for urgent radiotherapy and high-dose corticosteroids (dexamethasone 16–30 mg/day) to prevent paralysis and incontinence.

Radiotherapy is of value in the treatment of symptoms other than pain. Haemoptysis, haematuria, and rectal or vaginal bleeding usually respond to a short course of treatment, 25 Gy in 5 or 6 fractions. Local irradiation of a superficial tumour mass may often prevent fungation occurring. Once fungation has taken place, irradiation will often reduce tumour bulk and lessen discharge and bleeding.

Superior vena caval obstruction should be treated with corticosteroids and mediastinal irradiation if the patient is well enough. Cough, dyspnoea, and dysphagia caused by pressure from tumour will often respond to palliative radiotherapy.

Chemotherapy and hormonal manipulation have a minor place in the symptom control of the terminally ill, but they are worth considering for tumours which are chemosensitive or hormone dependent.

Anaesthetic techniques for pain control

The benefits of an anaesthetic procedure for the cancer patient will depend not only on the site and severity of pain but also on the availability of an anaesthetist specializing in this work who can carry it out with the minimum of delay or disturbance. At St. Christopher's Hospice, over the last years, the proportion of patients who have received such treatment has remained steady at 5–10 per cent, but the actual procedures have altered greatly.

In general, local anaesthetic and neurolytic conduction blockade of peripheral nerves and sympathetic ganglia are performed less often and epidural administration of local anaesthetics, opioids, and corticosteroids is more common. Transcutaneous electrical nerve stimulation (TENS) is occasionally useful for the control of cancer pain. Acupuncture has rarely been found to be effective. However, the field continues to change, so that close liaison with a local anaesthetist and pain clinic is essential. The chapter 'Anaesthetic techniques for pain control' in the *Oxford Textbook of Palliative Medicine* gives details of the procedures available (Swarm and Cousins 1993).

Adjuvant analgesic drugs

Certain cancer pains are relatively 'morphine insensitive' in that severe side-effects occur when the dose of morphine is increased and satisfactory pain control cannot be achieved. The correct use of adjuvants may occasionally mean that morphine is not required at all, more often it is possible to achieve better pain control, with a lower dose of morphine and fewer side-effects.

Unfortunately, the response to adjuvant analgesic drugs is very variable so that it is recommended that, unless delayed response is likely, the drug is discontinued after one or two weeks if there is no improvement. If this policy were widely followed, there would be fewer patients seen with intractable pain (usually neuropathic) who were receiving four or more adjuvant analgesic drugs but with no clear evidence which, if any, had helped.

Non-steroidal anti-inflammatory drugs (NSAIDs)

NSAIDs have anti-inflammatory, antipyretic, and analgesic properties. They can be used in the management of mild cancer pain, but paracetamol is usually preferred as it has fewer side-effects. Their main clinical use, in palliative care, is in the treatment of pain from bony metastases. Certain bone metastases liberate prostaglandins which sensitise nerve-endings to painful stimuli. NSAIDs inhibit prostaglandin biosynthesis. They are therefore peripherally acting analgesics, whereas opioids act centrally. While the main indication for these drugs is bone pain, they are also sometimes helpful in pelvic, liver, and cutaneous pain. There are no clinical trials comparing different NSAIDs in cancer pain, so it is better to become familiar with a few drugs chosen from different chemical classes. Unfortunately there is a considerable incidence of gastrointestinal toxicity and it may be wise to give concurrent misoprostol in susceptible patients, for example, those who are also receiving corticosteroids.

Antidepressant drugs

Antidepressant drugs have a specific analgesic effect in many types of chronic pain. This is independent of their effect on mood as it occurs more rapidly, at a lower dose and in the non-depressed patient.

The main indication for these drugs, as adjuvant analgesics, is in the patient with neuropathic pain. They are the first choice if the pain is described as 'burning' but can also be used for lancinating pain. The older tricyclic antidepressants seem the most effective, for example, amitriptyline 10–25 mg at night, increasing to 75–150 mg, as tolerated.

A proportion of cancer patients, with or without pain, become clinically depressed. They should be given anti-depressants and receive psychological help. As the depression lifts, quite frequently the complaint of pain lessens.

Anticonvulsant drugs

Carbamazepine is the anticonvulsant drug most commonly used as an adjuvant analgesic. Its main value is in the management of lancinating neuropathic pain, but it some-times helps the patient with continuous dysaesthesia. The usual starting dose is 200 mg daily, increasing up to 1000 mg daily in divided doses, depending on response and side-effects. Other anticonvulsant drugs such as sodium valproate, phenytoin, and clonazepam, have been similarly used for neuropathic pain.

Local anaesthetic drugs

The intravenous infusion of a local anaesthetic has been shown to relieve certain types of pain and these results have been repeated with oral local anaesthetics such as flecainide and mexilitine. Their main clinical use is in the management of neuropathic pain, the usual starting dose is flecanide 50 mg twice daily, increasing to 100 mg twice daily. These drugs should be avoided in patients with pre-existing ischaemic heart disease.

Corticosteroids

Corticosteroids have been used in a wide variety of types of cancer pain. Their main effect is probably caused by reducing inflammatory oedema around tumour masses and thus lessening the pressure on pain-sensitive structures. They may also reduce hyperexcitability in damaged nerves. Examples of steroid-responsive pain include headaches from raised intra-cranial pressure, epidural spinal cord compression, plexus or peripheral nerve infiltration or compression, bone pain, liver or pelvic pain. For severe pain, dexamethasone 16 mg daily is recommended, reducing the dose as possible. For mild pain much lower doses such as dexamethasone 4–6 mg daily can be used.

Other adjuvant analgesics

The phenothiazines, other than methotrimeprazine, have not been shown to have an analgesic effect. However, it is widely recognized that anxiety and tension increase the experience of pain and therefore drugs which lessen anxiety, such as halo-peridol or a benzodiazepine, will probably lessen pain in the anxious patient.

Diazepam or baclofen can be used to reduce painful muscle spasm. Hyoscine butylbromide is used for painful intestinal colic and oxybutynin for bladder or urethral spasm.

The bisphosphonates have been shown in some studies to relieve bone pain; further controlled trials are awaited.

Simple procedures

Painful lymphoedema, secondary to cancer, requires intens-ive treatment with massage, compression bandaging, and exercises. When the swelling is reduced, it is usually possible to fit an elastic compression sleeve or stocking.

The pain from fungating tumours can be relieved by regu-lar cleansing and soothing dressings. Catheterization will eliminate the painful and distressing frequency sometimes associated with bladder cancer.

Results of treatment

Experience from UK hospices shows that 85 per cent of cancer patients have pain satisfactorily and relatively easily controlled. A further 10 per cent prove more difficult, requiring frequent alterations of the drug regimen and perhaps non-drug methods to maintain control of pain. In the remaining 5 per cent pain control is not satisfactory. An analysis of these usually shows one or more of the following factors: severe, but intermittent pain; a short time or poor compliance with treatment; major emotional or family problems. These results have now been supported by many studies from all over the world. The foundation of these has been the WHO Guidelines with advice about the correct use of opioids and adjuvant analgesia. There is increased consumption of morphine for medical purposes in most countries and this must mean that many more patients are receiving the pain control that they need (WHO 1990). Yet in spite of these findings, patients still suffer unnecessarily and the following case can occur.

Mr H.G. aged 73, had palliative surgery for a carcinoma of stomach, followed over the next months by six courses of chemotherapy. He developed severe pain which was not relieved by the medication he received and, in desperation, he twice attempted to kill himself, first with an overdose of dextromoramide and later by slashing his wrists. On transfer to the hospice he said 'The pain was driving me crazy'.

His pain was controlled within 48 hours by oral morphine solution, 30 mg 4-hourly. His comment after 12 hours was 'last night's sleep was a gift'. The dose was gradually increased during the following three weeks to 60 mg 4-hourly. As soon as he was free from pain he no longer wished to end his life, but as the disease progressed he became increasingly weak and dyspnoeic. During his last few days he had occasional episodes of confusion, but was still able to walk to the toilet the day before he died.

This patient should have received adequate analgesia, or perhaps a coeliac plexus block, while he was having chemotherapy. His pain proved easy to control and he would then have had relief for the full nine months of his advancing illness and not merely during the final three weeks.

5

Control of symptoms
other than pain

The patient with terminal malignant disease usually presents a complex clinical picture. The tumour has often metastasized, resistance to infection may be reduced, renal and hepatic function impaired, and there is usually considerable debility. It is therefore not surprising that patients develop a multiplicity of symptoms in the last weeks or months of life. The foundation of good terminal care is meticulous attention to each symptom presented. Without this it is difficult, perhaps impossible, to give the necessary emotional support to the patient and family.

An analysis of the symptoms on admission to St. Christopher's Hospice in 1985 is shown in Table 2.

Palliative treatment involves making a diagnosis of the cause, or causes, of each symptom. For the patient who is terminally ill, this diagnosis will be based on a careful history and physical examination with the minimum of investigations. The information should be recorded using problem-orientated notes. For example: Mr S.L. (62). Squamous carcinoma of left bronchus. Dyspnoea due to tumour and large left pleural effusion, exacerbated by a chest infection and his increasing anxiety about the future.

Such a diagnosis will point to any reversible causes of the symptom. But even if the causes are irreversible, a knowledge of the mechanisms involved will indicate the correct symptomatic treatment.

The section that follows is a brief account of the diagnosis and treatment of some of the common symptoms found in

Table 2 Symptoms of 742 patients on admission to St. Christopher's Hospice in 1985

Symptom	Percentage		
	Total	Male	Female
Weakness	91	93	90
Weight loss	79	85	74
Anorexia	76	78	74
Pain	62	61	64
Dyspnoea	51	58	47
Constipation	51	56	47
Cough	45	60	33
Nausea/Vomiting	44	42	47
Dysphagia	25	28	22
Insomnia	24	25	24

terminal illness. For a fuller review of the subject see Suggestions for further reading (p. 61).

Anorexia

Causative factors such as hypercalcaemia, infection, and depression should be treated. Good mouth care is important and pain, nausea, and constipation require symptomatic treatment. Drug treatment includes corticosteroids, either dexamethasone 2–4 mg daily or prednisolone 15–30 mg daily, and high-dose progestagens, megestrol acetate 160 mg daily or medroxyprogesterone 300 mg daily.

Confusion

The differential diagnosis and treatment of confusion are two of the most difficult problems facing the doctor who is caring for dying patients. Whereas pain, or perhaps incontinence, is the symptom most dreaded by the patient, confusion is the symptom that most distresses the family.

It is important to seek a diagnosis of the cause (or causes) of confusion. Potentially reversible causes include medication, especially opioids and psychotropic drugs, infections, hypercalcaemia, and cerebral oedema.

Non-drug methods of management are always required; a familiar routine is helpful, if possible in home surroundings. The 'quietly muddled' patient requires no medication and sedative drugs may worsen things. Psychotropic drugs are, however, needed to reduce agitation, hallucinations, or paranoia. Haloperidol is usually effective and causes little sedation, thioridazine or chlorpromazine can be substituted, or diazepam added if sedation is required.

Constipation

The causes of constipation in the terminally ill are usually irreversible. They include inactivity, a diet low in roughage, general weakness, and the constipating effects of drugs such as opioids and tricyclic antidepressants.

Laxatives are the mainstay of treatment and should be prescribed routinely when starting opioids. They can be divided into those that primarily stimulate peristalsis such as senna, bisacodyl and danthron, and those whose main effect is to soften and bulk the stool, for example, magnesium hydroxide, lactulose, and poloxamer.

In clinical practice, a combination of both types of laxatives is the most effective. Examples include lactulose and bisacodyl, magnesium hydroxide and liquid paraffin emulsion with senna and codanthramer (danthron and poloxamer). The dose should be gradually increased until a regular soft bowel action is obtained. Suppositories or an enema or manual removal may be needed if a patient presents with a loaded rectum or if the laxative regimen is ineffective. It is a good general rule to perform a rectal examination on the third day if the bowels have not opened, inserting a glycerine or bisacodyl suppository if the rectum is loaded.

Cough

The cause of cough should be identified, if possible, and appropriate treatment offered. However, in many cases such treatment is not possible or is ineffective, and symptomatic treatment is required. In general terms it is reasonable to suppress a dry cough but a productive cough should be allowed to continue unless it is disturbing sleep or the patient is too weak to expectorate effectively. Treatment options include:

- Steam inhalations or nebulized saline aid the expectoration of viscid sputum.
- Simple linctus seems to soothe the pharynx and reduce coughing.
- Codeine linctus 10–20 ml (30–60 mg) 4–6 hourly.
- Morphine 5 mg 4-hourly, increasing the dose as necessary.
- Nebulized local anaesthetic, using 5 ml of 2% lignocaine, up to four times daily has sometimes been used with benefit.

Dysphagia

Difficulty in swallowing can be due to painful lesions, mechanical obstruction, or a neuromuscular disorder affecting the mouth, pharynx, or oesophagus. Patients with a dry mouth, anorexia, and anxiety may also complain of dysphagia. The following treatments are available:

- Thrush infection. Treatment is with nystatin or the systemic agents, ketoconazole or fluconazole.
- Oesophageal cancer. Depending on the histology and site, treatment with radiotherapy, laser therapy, bouginage or a flexible oesophageal tube may be indicated.
- Mediastinal lymphadenopathy. Radiotherapy should be considered, corticosteroids (dexamethasone 8 mg/day) sometimes give temporary relief.

Modification of the diet is needed so that the right consistency of food is served in an attractive form. A few patients, with slow growing and localized disease, benefit from the insertion of a fine bore nasogastric tube or a gastrostomy.

Dyspnoea

It is important to seek a diagnosis of the cause(s) of breathlessness for there are many potentially reversible factors. These include chest infection, cardiac failure, pleural effusion, superior vena caval obstruction, airways obstruction, and anxiety. In most patients, these should, in the first instance, be treated actively provided that the necessary symptomatic measures are used as well.

However, as the disease progresses, the place for active treatment becomes less and one or more of the following symptomatic treatments are needed:

- Explanation and adjustment.
- Oral morphine. The mechanism of action of morphine remains unclear but it appears to reduce the sensation of dyspnoea more than it reduces the level of ventilation. Clinical experience indicates that oral morphine, starting

at 2.5–5 mg 4-hourly and increasing slowly to 20 mg is safe and effective.

- Nebulized morphine. The usual starting dose is 10 mg. It can be given 4-hourly or used, when needed, before exercise.
- Diazepam 2–10 mg at night is used for its anxiolytic effect, sometimes in combination with morphine.
- Buspirone 5–10 mg 8-hourly is a less sedating anxiolytic drug.
- Hyoscine. This is used, in combination with diamorphine, to lessen the 'death rattle' which can occur in the last hours of life. The dose is 0.4 mg–0.6 mg 4-hourly by injection or up to 2.4 mg/day by subcutaneous infusion.
- Oxygen. The use of oxygen in the dyspnoea of terminal illness is controversial and the benefits do not correlate well with the level of oxygen saturation. Drug treatment for dyspnoea is recommended first, followed by a trial of oxygen if the dyspnoea remains severe.

Intestinal obstruction

Intestinal obstruction is a common complication of ovarian cancer. It occurs less often with colorectal cancer and can be caused by many other primary tumours. The obstruction may be mechanical or due to a motility disorder and may be present at many sites in both small and large bowel.

Palliative surgery should always be considered if the patient is well enough and wishes for it. Guidelines for this have been established. Gastrointestinal intubation and intravenous fluids are of value when a decision about surgery is made, but they should rarely be continued long-term (Baines 1993).

The majority of patients with inoperable intestinal obstruction can be managed well with pharmacological treatment. Drugs are mixed together and given by subcutaneous infusion using a portable syringe driver. Symptoms and treatment are as follows:

- Intestinal colic. Stimulant laxatives should be stopped. Diamorphine may be adequate but often hyoscine butylbromide 60–200 mg/day is needed.
- Continuous abdominal pain. Diamorphine subcutaneously, titrating the dose against response.
- Nausea and vomiting. Treatment is started with haloperidol 5–15 mg/day or cyclizine 150 mg/day. Hyoscine butylbromide can be added to reduce gastric secretions. An alternative is octreotide, a somatostatin analogue, 0.2–0.9 mg/day. This reduces gastrointestinal secretions and lessens vomits. Methotrimeprazine 50–200 mg/day is used for intractable vomiting, but causes sedation. Patients are allowed to eat and drink as they choose.

Nausea and vomiting

Vomiting results from impulses reaching the vomiting centre in the medulla. It can be stimulated from the chemoreceptor trigger zone, from afferent impulses from the gut, from the vestibular centre or directly due to raised intracranial pressure and from psychogenic causes. Thus there are a large number of potential causes of nausea and vomiting, originating in many parts of the body.

Nausea can often be treated with oral medication but a subcutaneous infusion of anti-emetic(s) is required for the management of severe vomiting. Common causes and recommended treatment are as follows:

- Opioid-induced vomiting. Metoclopramide should be given prophylactically.
- Uraemia. Haloperidol is usually effective.

- Hypercalcaemia. This is treated with intravenous rehydration and bisphosphonates.
- Gastric stasis. This can be caused by drugs, especially opioids, or by pressure from an enlarged liver or ascites. Metoclopramide is usually effective.
- Inoperable intestinal obstruction (see p. 40).
- Constipation (see p. 37).
- Raised intracranial pressure. Dexamethasone is the treatment of choice; if contraindicated, cyclizine is usually effective.
- Vestibular disturbance. Both cyclizine and hyoscine are used.
- Anxiety. Often a combination of psychological support and an anxiolytic drug is needed.

Sore mouth

A dry or painful mouth is common in those with terminal disease. Causes include drugs, thrush infection, dehydration, and poorly fitting dentures. Good oral hygiene is most important. Teeth and dentures should be cleaned regularly. Mouthwashes with chlorhexidine 0.2% or povidone iodine 1% both moisten and cleanse the mouth.

Thrush infections are common and should be treated with nystatin suspension or with the systemic antifungal drugs, fluconazole and ketoconazole.

Buccal analgesics include benzydamine (Difflam), a NSAID absorbed through the mucosa, and choline salicylate (Bonjela) which can be applied to painful or ulcerated areas.

The last days

The correct management of the last few days of life involves the care of both patient and family. The way in which the death is handled will influence the family's grief, bereavement, and their ability to cope with the future. Those who visit the bereaved will be only too aware how the last few hours become imprinted on the memory with unanswerable questions: 'I wonder if she was trying to say something to me?', 'Do you think he was in pain?'

As death approaches there is usually a gradual increase in drowsiness and weakness, and it is often the experienced nurse who will recognize that this is not a temporary deterioration but represents the imminence of death. The 'diagnosis of dying' needs to be confirmed by the doctor who should then review the medication stopping all drugs except those for symptom relief. Drugs to withdraw include antibiotics, diuretics, antihypertensives, and laxatives. Corticosteroids and NSAIDs are usually continued until the patient cannot swallow.

Studies have shown that two-thirds of patients continue to take some oral medication until the last day of life. However, essential drugs must be charted so that, if swallowing becomes impossible, they can be given by injection, subcutaneous infusion, or suppository. In the home, this will involve having the required drugs immediately available and written-up by the attending doctor. The essential drugs are as follows:

- Diamorphine or morphine. The oral dose should be converted to the dose for injection and given either by subcutaneous infusion or 4-hourly (p. 22).

- Anticonvulsants should be replaced by diazepam suppositories 10–20 mg twice daily or midazolam by subcutaneous infusion.

- Hyoscine hydrobromide 0.4 mg–0.6 mg 4-hourly or up to 2.4 mg/day by subcutaneous infusion may be needed to relieve the 'Death rattle'.

- Psychotropic drugs. While most patients become more drowsy and lapse into coma as death approaches, some become restless and agitated. This may be due to unrelieved pain or a distended bladder or rectum but frequently no cause can be identified. Benzodiazepines (diazepam and midazolam), phenothiazines, and phenobarbitone have proved effective in this situation. Suggested doses are:

Diazepam suppositories 10–20 mg 8-hourly.

Midazolam 30–100 mg/day by subcutaneous infusion.

Methotrimeprazine 25–50 mg 4–8 hourly or by subcutaneous infusion.

Chlorpromazine, up to 300 mg/day can be given by suppository or intramuscular injection. It is too irritant to use subcutaneously.

Phenobarbitone, 200–600 mg/day by subcutaneous infusion. A separate syringe driver will be needed as it cannot be mixed with other drugs.

Medication, although important, is not the only way of managing a restless dying patient. Staff often notice that the presence of the family or nurse sitting by the bedside, holding the hand, or speaking quietly to an apparently unconscious patient has a remarkably calming effect.

6

Other components of total pain

As we understand better the physical aspects of terminal care, we find more subtle and complex problems to tackle. In the same way, as we face the totality of a patient's suffering we begin to understand more about its mental, social, and spiritual components and often find similar complexity. Where physical pain remains difficult to control these must be explored and although such division may be somewhat artificial it will enlighten us as we endeavour to understand the suffering of each patient and to help both them and their families.

The use of the word 'pain' must not trap us into thinking that it demands the immediate use of appropriate drugs. This pain should usually be faced rather than merely blotted out. There is often hard work to be done in this time of crisis and sometimes only the facing of the deepest issues in anguish will enable the patient to accept what is happening in terms of his own identity and aims, and the family to find the strengths that will help them to face the future. Surprising growth can be achieved in a short time, as in all situations of crisis.

Mental pain

It is still rare to find, among the results of the investigations and examinations with which a patient's notes are filled, any comment on feelings or an estimation of insight into what is happening. These may well be the main problems, greatly exacerbating the total pain and undermining the capacity to cope with increasing weakness. Any illness causes anxiety, especially one that becomes more serious despite a variety of treatments until it is patently life threatening. Many patients still tend to be left alone with their fears or only receive reassurances which they suspect are false. Mental suffering is likely to be enhanced by any physical distress; the doctor can do much to relieve the one as the other is tackled. Discussion of palliative treatments and competent symptom control can open up communication and bring support at a deep level, demanding time with the patient and the close contact often denied at this stage. Isolation adds to all suffering, particularly to the feeling of failure and the sense of guilt suffered by many dying patients. Sensitive honesty engenders trust and can be supportive to both patient and family. The question of truth, of how to break bad news, is frequently discussed. However, no report can take the place of an attentive listening and response to the questions an individual patient is asking at a particular time.

Only a minority of patients are likely to have a history of psychiatric or emotional disorder, but it is important to discover this at the first history taking. These patients may not need special help, but difficulties will at least be easier to understand. Nearly all will be helped by a chance to talk of their feelings with a sympathetic listener, and while only a few will need the help of a psychiatrist, all of us can learn by discussing their reactions both with psychiatrists and with social workers. Their role may be found in such consultations, as they meet the patient at 'second hand', but in our experience ward meetings in which they are involved will encourage all the staff to develop their own confidence and expertise and to refer those who need extra skills.

Those who have had the opportunity to listen constantly to dying people recognize they may show a variety of reactions. Kubler-Ross (1970) described these as stages of realization and Parkes (1984) compared them with the progress through bereavement and other forms of loss. Both writers emphasize that some of these stages may be omitted, that they may not occur in clear-cut order, may overlap, or may be gone through more than once, particularly in an illness that has remissions and relapses or a series of progressive deteriorations. Any attempt to impose a kind of blueprint would be wrong but many of us have seen our patients make a journey and we can often expect progress and hope for adjustment to what is happening. Most human beings have the capacity for coming to terms with their circumstances, which they retain even as death approaches, though for some it is a struggle that is deeply painful to watch. Others appear to hold quite contradictory feelings in an uneasy balance.

Anyone who is faced with disaster or bad news tends to react initially with disbelief or denial. This is difficult to sustain and as it begins to waver a patient may display yearning and protest similar to the restless pining of early bereavement. They may feel angry about what is happening to them and project this on to their treatment and those who gave it to them, to their families, and to fate: 'I was all right until I had radiotherapy'; 'The operation went wrong'; 'It's your pills, doctor'. Similar feelings are often present in the family who are facing bereavement, who may also defend themselves from its pain by projecting their anger on to the staff. These are feelings which can be worked through if they can be expressed to people who understand something of the reason for them and do not react by offended silence or withdrawal. It is at this point that the help of a social worker or psychiatrist as back-up to the ward team can be particularly helpful.

Another 'stage' is reached when a patient appears to give up hope, turns the anger inward, and lapses into depression and despair. Such people only rarely contemplate suicide but those around often fear this and boost hope again, however unjustified this may be. This inhibits further progress towards adjustment. This phase is perhaps best regarded as sadness—a natural reaction—more often than as clinical depression. Used with discrimination, antidepressant drugs sometimes help but the listener who understands and is not overwhelmed by the situation helps most of all.

Many people can and do work their way through all these reactions. This has been described as a 'last stage' of acceptance and our experience would endorse this. People can come to accept death as inevitable, although a faint hope of an unexpected recovery against all expectations may remain at the same time. Hope can exist in different forms throughout such an illness, gradually changing in content. The small day-by-day hopes help the patient to accept the responsibility of living the life that remains. The quality of such living and the maturity of someone who has reached this acceptance is seen by many in this field as the most powerful argument against any deliberate shortening of life. So many emotional and interpersonal problems seem only to be solved at the very end.

There are no hard rules. Some fortunate people seem able to make this journey with simplicity and scarcely any of the anguish and fears that can be overwhelming. Their sadness at parting is comforted by the love and friendship of those around and they continue to give back the same. Others go through the whole process in one or two intense sessions and then take each day as it comes, perhaps never discussing the matter again, like the man who said 'I've had it all out with my wife, now we can relax and talk about something else'.

Just as hope may continue in a different guise throughout an illness, so too may fear. Fears of parting, of what will happen to dependants, of pain and weakness, of the whole mystery of death, and of failing to cope are all common among dying patients. Although the complexity of the problems faced by many are daunting, it need not make us feel helpless. Dying is not a psychiatric illness and does not usually call for specialized skills in counselling in depth. Those who distance themselves, feeling that they can bring nothing but a lack of comprehension, do not realize that it is often their attempt to understand and not success in doing so that eases the patient's loneliness. Their own feelings of helplessness bring them to patients at their level and here they can help with silence more than with words. The person who came nearest to helping the dying Ivan Illich as he struggled through his anguished queries about the meaning of life was the peasant boy who willingly stayed physically near to him (Tolstoy 1887).

Nurses are usually closer to their patients than doctors and are likely to hear more of the questions and fears. Team consultations are essential if we are to reach a helpful understanding. The social worker or chaplain can listen in a unique way, for they are not involved with physical therapy and are experienced as the recipients of unacceptable feelings and projected angers. Negative feelings in this situation may be frighteningly strong and these are better expressed than buried only to appear in a different guise, often affecting both family and staff. Time with physiotherapists offers more than the pleasure of assisted movements or even the joy of tackling the stairs again with the consequent reward of the weekend home. It is well known that the interested ward orderly may hear more than anyone of matters which a patient is unable to share with the professionals who surround him. We must not forget that boredom may be a major component of mental pain and a good gossip, like other distractions, are good ways to relieve it. Imaginative occupational therapy and any chance to be creative are healing to such feelings; so too may be the contact with the group in a department separate from the ward. Many units have developed imaginative Day Centres and seen unexpected transformations.

The distinction between mental and social pain may be hard to sustain—for much of a patient's fears concern his family. Some of those we care for will be loners who are usually remarkably philosophical about dying, leaving no responsibilities, but for the majority we must widen our concern to family and close friends.

Social pain

When an illness has a foreseeable end it is still true that many families will come to grips with the situation and will wish to look after a dying relative at home for as long as possible. Although the trend has been for a higher proportion of cancer deaths to occur in hospital, prolongation of life by the newer treatments often means that much of this extra time is spent at home and the present approach is to enable a patient to stay home (usually the preferred place) until the end. Only a minority will require heavy nursing for any length of time but there may be a prolonged period of emotional strain for patient and family alike. If they can be helped to handle this it may be an important time for them all, for it enables the survivors to complete any 'unfinished business'. Old tensions may become acute but even at this stage, often because it *is* the final stage, reconciliation is not uncommon and many people make this a remarkably fruitful time. People in crisis often show an astonishing ability to resolve long-standing problems and even to handle new ones. The family, like the patient, have a journey to travel and much patience and support may be needed as they battle their way through.

Time spent with the family on first seeing or soon after the giving of a poor prognosis will help to establish or reaffirm trust and confidence. Explanations of the probable progress of the disease, of what can be done to control pain and other likely symptoms, and some discussions of the actual process of dying will be needed. People have frightening images of dying and the increasing dependence and physical changes in some dying patients may serve to enhance them. Yet it has been shown in many settings that with competent care almost all patients with terminal cancer will sink quietly into unconsciousness and die peacefully. Families are unlikely to know this unless we tell them and may live with unnecessary fears to worsen their sorrow and natural apprehension. Other practical reassurances may be needed, for example, who to contact in a crisis; how much to expect of a visiting nurse, a home help, or a night sitter; and what aids or supplementary benefits may be obtainable.

Children and adolescents should be involved. Attempts to protect them are usually counter-productive and they are deeply hurt if they are excluded. They need explanations of the disease and its treatment that the patient is unlikely to be able to give them, as well as reassurance that cancer is neither contagious nor hereditary. Discussions with whole families, including the children and often the patient, have gradually become more common in St. Christopher's Hospice. The Social Work Department has facilitated this but a doctor or senior nurse who can give time for unlimited listening can handle many such situations given the support of the rest of the ward team. This may not be easy in either a busy practice or an acute ward and the growth of specialized hospital or home care teams who will work alongside regular staff can bring extra time and experience where the latter are hard pressed.

Patients who are kept in the dark about family finances and various practical matters will have the added burden of fancying they have hurt or offended others because of the barriers thus erected. Financial burdens are often heavy, especially for those who have prolonged time off work, but patients should be included in all discussions and plans, as they should be involved as far as possible in ordinary family life. One can understand the strong desire to keep all worries from the patient, yet this protectiveness often leads to crippling tensions and it is sad since the patient is likely to come to know the truth by other means. To keep an unshared secret from a close friend inevitably impairs communication and can add greatly to the general distress.

We have also found that many couples are greatly relieved when they are encouraged slowly to share as much of the truth as they seem able to handle. Family relationships are often complex and disturbed but although some will demand much help from a social worker it is surprising how many will battle their own way through with the care and support of their usual doctors and nurses.

If admission to hospital or hospice becomes necessary, it may bring comfort for the patient and reduction of anxiety for the family but these must not be brought at the cost of feelings of guilt. The family must be reassured that they have done what they could and that professional help is now needed on a full-time basis. The ward staff must not take over care in such a way as to exclude the family, who may not easily be involved with the physical care of the patient. When possible this should be encouraged but they can contribute greatly to security and peace by their mere presence and this should certainly be made both possible and explicit. Family have a right to be present at this time, both cared for and caring, and their unique role must be emphasized and re-inforced. The social worker and the chaplain may still be much involved with those who react aggressively to their pain or are overwhelmed by their feelings, but every member of staff should be able to give some recognition, even if brief, to the family that is maintaining its last watch with a dying member.

The long pain of the family's bereavement is a part of terminal pain. They will begin to grieve their imminent parting during the illness but the real letting go and approach to the new situation will rarely happen before the patient dies. The final watch and the witnessing of a peaceful death may be very important for some families; others cannot remain by the bedside. Staying there may not be possible or advisable, and care must be taken to protect them from feelings of guilt and responsibility. Ward staff are all too familiar with the desolation of the final moment of parting and the empty numbness that follows it but do not always appreciate how greatly their supporting presence can help, both then and when the family returns afterwards.

An increasing number of units and teams in the Hospice and Palliative Care Movement have included bereavement follow-up work and they attempt to identify those families who appear to need extra support in the initial stages of their life without the patient. More work needs to be done in this field both in selecting those who need help and in understanding how best to give it. The social worker may well be in contact with such a family before the patient dies but the ward team should report unusually disturbed or disturbing behaviour. Some people from cultures different from our own may show noisy expression of grief, which must somehow be allowed without upsetting an entire ward. An inability to show any emotion is usually a poor prognostic sign.

Some families ask for sedatives but this is probably mistaken. Grief needs to be expressed at this point and drugs may inhibit this natural and eventually healing reaction. There is no ground for prescribing tranquillizers or antidepressants to the bereaved as a routine. Parkes (1984) believes that such drugs should be reserved for the potentially suicidal, for whom a referral to expert help may be needed in emergency. Such drugs may be needed by those who, despite all efforts to help, remain in a state of chronic agitation or depression. A mild hypnotic may be needed for those whose sleep remains disturbed but can easily become habit forming.

The bereaved family comes slowly to full realization of what has happened and after often intense inner struggle and dejection is eventually ready to build a new life. This may take many months and is felt like a sort of illness which is finally healed. Abnormal, unresolved grief needs skilled help.

The whole process of bereavement is not often seen by clinicians other than family doctors but all of us should accept two responsibilities. Firstly, to see that others are alert to identifying and helping those who are especially at risk in their loss; and secondly, to do all that they can to ease the memories of those who live on by giving the best possible relief of terminal distress.

Most dying people show remarkable endurance and those who spend their time close to them find that this helps to reduce their own fears of death. Most of the dying have a good heritage to leave, which is not always recognized or received either by the staff around them or, more important, by the family themselves. The bereaved too have much to hand on. Parkes writes of his admiration for many of the people who have shared their grief with him and finds that counselling them has made it easier to recognize bereavement as an acceptable part of life (Parkes 1984).

Spiritual pain

Few people today are likely to express their doubts and griefs in terms that are recognizably religious. Nevertheless, feelings of failure and regret—'If only . . .'; 'I wish I hadn't . . .'; 'It's too late.'—are all common and often intense. Many patients need help to face feelings of guilt and worthlessness that can truly be described as spiritual pain, sometimes amounting to deep anguish. This becomes apparent as we listen, however much the spiritual component may seem to be swamped by difficulties of personality, culture, or past history. Some have a background of religious affiliation and early liaison with or through the chaplain in hospital or with the priest or minister of the patient's own choice at home may be important. His ability to pronounce the forgiveness that always awaits every man can be manifestly healing. Others have no such starting place but we have seen how an atmosphere of acceptance created by a whole ward team or by an individual member visiting in a home can reach and assuage such pain.

Our own religious or philosophical convictions can help in creating such a climate but it is no precondition of effective help that a patient should accept these beliefs and each one must be so free of any pressure to conform that the thought never enters the mind. There is a progression from trust in the acceptance by others of all the things in ourselves that we regret into a faith in forgiveness, where we at last believe that they have no more power to hurt us or anyone else. We cannot alter what has happened or what we have done, but we can come to believe that the meaning of the past can be changed. From this comes the ability to forgive ourselves. This may never be expressed in words on either side but the quality of the ensuing peace is unmistakable.

A feeling of meaningless, that neither oneself nor the universe itself has permanence or purpose, is a form of spiritual pain. Patients need to look back over the story of their lives and believe that there was some sense in them and also to reach out towards something greater than themselves, a truth to which they can be committed. This is often linked with the belief that somehow life goes on: 'In all of us the archaic belief in the immortality of the soul is still dormant' (Eissler 1955); 'As anyone who has done much pastoral or counselling work will know, the belief (or perhaps it would often be better described as a feeling or intuition) that our visible, physical life is not the whole of our personal history is exceptionally tenacious' (Baker 1981). Eissler was sure that this belief, although it had no place in his scientific frame of reference, was present in both the patient and himself and should be used to help lift the burden of grief until the patient finally lost consciousness. Baker, holding the conviction that 'God can and will re-create our being even beyond annihilation', looked beyond to another dimension where the individual's capacity to love and worship will be fulfilled in freedom. We meet some who seem to have had little chance of a worthwhile life or death and find that our belief in a God who has himself gone through the rejection and death of a world of random pain and catastrophe keeps us close to such people with trust and hope for them.

Those hospices and homes that have some form of religious foundation will never care for more than a minority of all dying patients. Most will continue to die in their own homes or hospital wards where awareness of these issues is not normally seen as part of the care of the team as a whole. Here, the ward sister is likely to be the person with whom the chaplain has most to do, but some contact with a doctor may be essential. Consultation concerning the patient's needs and some idea of prognosis is required rather than detailed medical information, and this is likely to be most effective when it is informal and continuing. It would be unwarranted intrusion to suggest a contact when there is no understanding or willingness on the part of a patient and his family, but a chaplain who makes himself informally available is often surprised at his welcome. The gap that exists between the ordained ministry and the rest of us is not as wide as many believe it to be.

But we cannot leave it all to the chaplain, who in any case is often greatly overworked. Whoever we are and whatever our beliefs or lack of them we may have to face questions from the families and the patients and have to find the strength to listen when we feel we have no answers to give. The comment 'It makes you think' may be a plea for such listening at that moment from the person to whom it is addressed. The command 'Watch with me' did not mean 'Take this crisis away'; it could not have meant 'Explain it'; the simple, yet costly demand was 'Stay there and stay awake'. More of those who try to do this than will perhaps care to admit it will find themselves trusting in a Presence that can more easily reach the patient and the family if they themselves concentrate on using all their competence with compassion and say little to interrupt.

Staff pain

The staff themselves often need support, especially during their first weeks in terminal care. This work causes pain and bewilderment at times to all in this field and the closer the staff are to the weakness of the patients and the grief of the families the more they too will suffer the pangs of bereavement.

Nurses meeting death for the first time find it awe inspiring, even uncanny, and they and their colleagues in general wards are likely to question whether they did everything they should have done. They often feel overwhelmed and need an early opportunity to discuss this with someone more senior, preferably someone who has also known the patient. Those who choose to work in hospices are far more likely now than even 10 years ago to have had this opportunity during their general training and to have seen enough of what can be achieved in an acute ward to want to learn and then develop this in their turn.

Doctors are not immune to such feelings and are perhaps even more likely to question whether in fact the death was not due to a failure on their part. They may have had opportunity for discussion as students but, even so, the first death after they have qualified and have some responsibility may be unexpectedly traumatic.

Staff members of all disciplines may find themselves suffering a process of bereavement, of loneliness and exhaustion, protest, anger, and depression, and will need to share this if they are to find their way through. Merely to deny or repress such feelings hinders any progress in dealing with themselves and hence with others in the future. The resilience of those who choose and continue to work exclusively in this field is won by a full understanding of what is happening and not by a retreat behind a technique. The initial impact of hospice or palliative or continuing care, at first hand, and the draining effect of its continual losses calls for some form of team or group support. This may well need to be varied; a series of group discussions seems to have a natural term and later another approach is needed. Spontaneous meetings (often as part of a ward report) that arise among those closely involved as a team continue to offer the most reliable as well as the most prompt and pertinent support. Those who are working in isolation need to find an understanding listener somehow.

Efficiency is always comforting. The giving of effective relief to all types of pain makes this an extremely rewarding field and, in itself, is a major form of support. Nevertheless, if we are to remain for long near the suffering of dependence and parting we need also to develop a basic philosophy and search, often painfully, for meaning in even the most adverse situations. We may be working with long and sometimes distressing physical retreats but these are so often more than balanced by emotional and spiritual advances. It is not idealistic to say that achievements are constantly being made during this time. From the dying themselves we learn not only to understand something of the ending of life but also a great deal to make us optimistic about all life and about the potential of those ordinary human beings who work their way through it.

We have to gain enough confidence in what we are doing and enough freedom from our anxieties to listen to another's distress. Only if we are prepared to do this will we find that most rewarding of all the aspects of terminal treatment and care: we will continue to know people at their most mature and their most courageous.

References

Baines, M.J. (1993). The pathophysiology and management of malignant intestinal obstruction. In *Oxford textbook of palliative medicine* (ed. D. Doyle, G.W.C. Hanks, and N. MacDonald), pp. 311–16.

Baker, J.A. (1981). A philosophy for dying. In *Hospice—the living idea* (ed. C. Saunders, D. Summers, and N. Teller), p. 68. Edward Arnold, London.

BMA (1988). *Euthanasia—Report of the Working Party to review the British Medical Association's Guidance on Euthanasia.* BMA, London.

Council of Europe (1976). *Recommendation 779 on the Rights of the sick and dying.* 27th Ordinary Session, January.

Devlin, P. (1985). *Easing the passing. The trial of Dr. John Bodkin Adams.* p. 171. The Bodley Head, London.

Eissler, K.R. (1955). *The psychiatrist and the dying patient,* p. 142. International Universities Press, New York.

House of Lords Report of the Select Committee on Medical Ethics (1994). HMSO, London.

Kubler-Ross, E. (1970). *On death and dying.* Tavistock Publications, London.

Lancet (1980). In cancer, honesty is here to stay. *Lancet,* ii, 245.

O'Brien, T., Kelly, M., and Saunders, C. (1992). Motor neurone disease—a hospice perspective. *British Medical Journal,* 304, 471–3.

Parkes, C.M. and Parkes, J. (1984). 'Hospice' versus 'Hospital' care—reevaluation after 10 years as seen by surviving spouses. *Postgraduate Medical Journal,* 60, 120.

Parkes, C.M. (1984). Psychological aspects. In *The management of terminal disease* (ed. C. Saunders). Edward Arnold, London.

Pius, XII, Pope (1957). *Acta Apostolicae Sedia,* 49, 1027.

Price, P., Hoskin, P.J., Easton, D., Austin, S., Palmer, S.G., and Yarnold, J.R. (1986). Prospective randomised trial of single and multifraction radiotherapy schedules in the treatment of painful bony metastases. *Radiotherapeutic Oncology,* 6, 247–55.

Swarm, R.A. and Cousins, M.J. (1993). Anaesthetic techniques for pain control. In *The Oxford textbook of palliative medicine* (ed. D. Doyle, G.W.C. Hanks, and N. MacDonald), pp. 204–21.

Tolstoy, L. (1887). *Ivan Illych*. Oxford University Press, Oxford.

World Health Organization (1990). *Cancer pain relief and palliative care*. WHO, Geneva.

Suggestions for further reading

Billings, J.A. (ed.) (1985). *The outpatient management of advanced cancer.* J. B. Lippincotte, Philadelphia.

Doyle, D., Hanks, G.W.C., and MacDonald, N. (eds) (1993). *Oxford textbook of palliative medicine.* Oxford University Press.

Saunders, C. (ed.) (1990). *Hospice and palliative care—an interdisciplinary approach.* Edward Arnold, London.

Saunders, C. and Sykes, N. (eds) (1993). *The management of terminal malignant disease*, (3rd edn). Edward Arnold, London.

Stedeford, A. (1984). *Facing death—patients, families, and professionals.* Heinemann, London.

Wall, P.D. and Melzack, R. (1994). *Textbook of pain*, (3rd edn). Churchill Livingstone, London.

Journals of interest

Palliative Medicine. Edward Arnold, London. A quarterly journal.

Journal of Pain and Symptom Management. Elsevier, Published eight times a year.

Index